A COMPASSIONATE GUIDE
TO PET LOSS

Navigating Grief and Healing After the Loss of a Beloved Pet Companion

Dedication

This book is born from the hearts of Jodi, Gary, and the Caregiver Brilliance team, each of us having walked the path of pet loss and grief.

We are deeply grateful for the opportunity to channel our own experiences into something that can offer comfort and guidance to others who may be suffering in silence. It is our hope that this book serves as a practical and tactile resource, encouraging personal reflection and meaningful conversations.

Our pets—dogs, cats, mice, and more—have shaped us into more compassionate human beings, and we dedicate this book to them. Their unconditional love has taught us the true meaning of connection and empathy.

In the spirit of Data, George, and our entire menagerie....

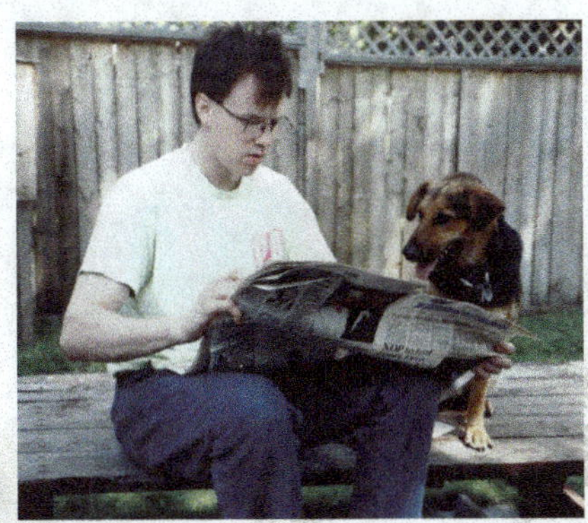

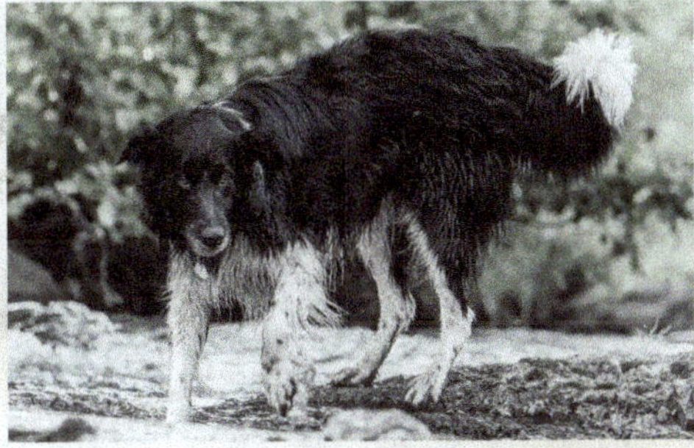

TABLE OF CONTENTS

A Gentle Invitation

Whether you are anticipating the loss of a beloved pet, grieving a recent departure, or revisiting a loss from long ago, this book will guide you through the tender emotions.

Pet Loss Guide: Healing From the Loss of A Beloved Pet is a self-guided reflective book designed to support you in your journey, offering comfort, understanding, and gentle healing for the raw emotions left by sadness following the death of a pet.

Pets often become cherished members of our families, and their loss can be as profound as losing a human loved one. The grief that follows can be complex and deeply felt. it's important to give yourself the space and time to heal.

This book is a companion inviting you to reflect, remember, and heal in a way that feels right for you. As you journey through these pages, take the initiative to journal your thoughts and feelings as they come—write directly in the book, respond to the questions, and use the extra pages at the end to explore your emotions further.

Through these reflections, may you find solace in your memories, strength in your emotions, and a gentle path toward healing.

The Stages of Grief:
Through the Lens of Pet Loss

Grief is the natural response to losing someone or something you love, and it's something everyone experiences differently.

Similarly, when you lose a pet, you may experience the same stages of grief. The stages, originally identified by Elizabeth Kubler Ross in 1969, are still widely recognized today as hallmarks of the grief cycle. It is important to note that these stages may repeat, or occur in a different order. And, there is no prescribed amount of time to spend in each stage.

Here's a simple way to understand these stages:

The Stages of Grief:
Through the Lens of Pet Loss

Denial "This Can't Be Happening"
What it is: It's hard to believe that your pet is really gone.
You might feel numb or in shock like the loss isn't real.
How it might feel: You might catch yourself expecting your
pet to come running around the corner or feel like you're
in a bad dream that you'll wake up from. This stage is your
mind's way of protecting you from the full impact of the
loss all at once.

Anger "Why Did This Happen?"
What it is: Anger is a natural reaction to feeling helpless or
unfairly treated by the situation. You might feel angry at
yourself, others, or even your pet for leaving you.
How it might feel: You might be upset with the vet, angry
at people who don't seem to understand your pain, or mad
that your pet got sick or had an accident. This stage is
about processing the deep hurt you feel.

The Stages of Grief:
Through the Lens of Pet Loss

Bargaining "If Only..."

What it is: You might start thinking about "what if" or "if only" scenarios. It's a way of trying to regain control or make sense of what happened.

How it might feel: You might think, "If only I had taken them to the vet sooner," or "What if I had done something different?" This stage is often filled with regret or guilt, even though most of these thoughts are based on things you couldn't control.

Depression "This Hurts So Much"

What it is: Depression in grief isn't just about feeling sad; it's a deep sense of loss and emptiness. It's when the reality of your pet's absence truly sinks in.

How it might feel: You might feel like there's a huge hole in your life where your pet used to be. This stage can be the hardest, but it's also a time when healing starts to happen, even if it doesn't feel like it yet.

The Stages of Grief:
Through the Lens of Pet Loss

Acceptance "I Miss Them, But I'm Okay"
What it is: Acceptance doesn't mean you're over the loss, but you've begun to find a way to live with it. You acknowledge that your pet is gone, and while it still hurts, you start to move forward.
How it might feel: You might begin to think about your pet with a smile rather than just sadness. Memories become a source of comfort, and you start to adjust to life without them physically by your side.

Being aware of the stages of grief, for a person or pet death, is a way of understanding and coping with the tsunami of emotions that you may be feeling.

Grief Triggers

Even after you've gone through the stages of grief, certain things can trigger those feelings of loss all over again. These "grief triggers" can be anything that reminds you of your pet.

Take some time and consider what are particularly painful reminders for you, and what changes you can make while you explore and heal these weighty grief emotions. By preparing yourself and anticipating the tender feelings, you can better navigate your life without denying your own emotional needs.

Common Grief Triggers

Seeing Other Pets:
Whether it's a pet that looks like yours or just seeing someone else with their pet, it can remind you of what you've lost.

Anniversaries:
Dates like your pet's birthday or the day they passed away can bring back strong emotions.

Routine Reminders:
Simple things, like feeding time or a favourite walking path, can trigger memories and sadness.

Managing Grief Triggers

Acknowledge the Trigger:

Recognizing that something has triggered your grief can help you take control of how you respond. It's okay to feel sad or upset—those feelings are a part of healing.

Find Comfort:

Have a go-to comfort activity for when these triggers happen, like writing in a journal, talking to someone who understands, or spending time in a place that brings you peace.

Create New Routines:

Slowly adapting your routine to one that doesn't focus on your pet can help lessen the impact of these triggers over time. This doesn't mean forgetting your pet but finding ways to move forward while still honouring their memory.

Dealing with Insensitivity

Dealing with insensitivity from others who don't value pets in the same way can be challenging. Unfortunately, not everyone understands the deep bond we form with our animal companions.

Sometimes, people might say things that feel hurtful, even if they don't mean to. They might think it's "just a pet" and not understand why you're so upset. It can be disheartening when our grief is dismissed or minimized.

Your grief is valid.

Finding comfort in others who have experienced a similar loss can be a welcome relief. If you encounter insensitivity, kindly express your need for support and understanding. Online pet loss communities can provide a safe space for connecting with people who truly understand.

It's okay to set boundaries and protect your emotional well-being. While it may be disheartening, remember that the love and bond you shared with your pet remain significant, regardless of how others perceive it.

Dealing with Insensitivity

Grieving the loss of a pet is deeply personal, not everyone will understand the depth of your emotions. Some people, even those who care about you, might make insensitive comments or fail to recognize your grief.

This activity will support you to reflect on how to interact with others during this time and to cope with insensitivity without hiding your emotions in a painful way.

A gentle reminder:

You Are Not Alone: Even if others don't understand, your feelings are valid. Seek out those who do understand.

It's Okay to Educate: Sometimes, a gentle explanation can help others see your perspective and become more empathetic.

Prioritize Your Well-being: Protect your emotional health by choosing carefully who you share your grief with and by setting boundaries when necessary.

Understand Their Perspective

Reflect: Consider that some people may not have experienced the deep bond that can exist between a person and their pet. They may not understand why you're grieving so deeply.

- Have I considered that this person might not fully understand the bond I had with my pet?
- How can I explain my feelings in a way that might help them understand?
- Is it possible that their insensitivity is unintentional or comes from a place of ignorance rather than malice?

Assess the Relationship

Reflect: Think about your relationship with the person who made the insensitive comment. How important is their opinion to you? How often do you interact with them?

- How significant is this person's opinion to my well-being?
- Do I interact with them regularly, or is this a one-time encounter?
- How much energy do I want to invest in explaining my feelings to them?

<u>Set Boundaries</u>
Reflect: It's okay to protect your emotional well-being by setting boundaries. Decide how much you want to share and with whom.
- What boundaries can I set to protect my emotions when interacting with this person?
- How can I politely but firmly express that their comments are hurtful?
- Would it be helpful to change the subject or divert the conversation when they bring up my loss?

Choose Your Support Circle

Reflect: Not everyone needs to be part of your grieving process. Choose to share your emotions with those who are empathetic and supportive.

- Who are the people in my life that truly understand and support me during this time?
- Are there certain people I should avoid discussing my grief with?
- How can I create a safe space where I can express my feelings freely and without judgment?

<u>Plan for Insensitive Interactions</u>

Reflect: Think ahead about how you might handle future interactions with insensitive individuals. Having a plan can help you feel more in control, encouraging a thoughtful response rather than an impulsive reaction.

- What will I say if someone makes an insensitive comment about my grief?
- Do I need a backup plan or someone to support me in these situations?
- How can I prepare myself emotionally before attending social events or gatherings where such comments might occur?

Unique Nature of Pet Grief

Grieving a pet is a deeply personal experience, different in many ways from grieving a human loved one. Pets offer us unconditional love, companionship, and a comforting presence in our daily lives. When they pass away, it's not just the loss of a friend but also the loss of routines and the emotional support they provided. This unique bond can leave a profound void that's hard for others to understand.

Pet grief is often misunderstood or overlooked, making it even more challenging to navigate. Without the same level of societal recognition as human loss, it can feel isolating and more difficult to process.

The next activity will help you reflect on these unique aspects of pet grief. Your responses will help you to better understand your loss and the special place your pet held in your life, guiding you toward healing.

Unique Nature of Pet Grief

Awareness of the Significance of Pet Loss
People recognize the loss of a pet as a significant event that can cause deep emotional pain. Society has become more understanding and accepting of pet owners' grief when their furry companions pass away.

Remember Individual Differences
Grief is a personal experience. People react differently to loss—some may experience intense sadness, while others might experience a mix of emotions, including guilt, anger, or even relief, particularly if the pet had been suffering from an illness.

Find Supportive Communities
Pet owners often find solace and support in online communities, forums, or social media groups dedicated to pet loss and grief. These platforms provide a space where individuals can share and receive empathy and understanding from others who truly understand.

Unique Nature of Pet Grief

Establish Rituals & Memorials

Holding funeral or memorial ceremonies, creating pet memorials, or participating in activities such as planting a tree or making a donation in the pet's name have become more common. Rituals help honour and remember the beloved companion while also providing a sense of closure.

Consider Professional Support

Some people may seek the assistance of pet loss counsellors or therapists who specialize in grief counselling. Professionals offer guidance and support during the grieving process, helping individuals navigate their emotions and find healthy coping strategies.

Additional Options

Some veterinary clinics offer home care services including End-of-Life care offering a serene alternative to a traditional clinic visit. Ask if they offer paw prints or hair clippings to keep as a memorial of your pet.

<u>Unconditional Love and Dependence:</u>

Pets offer unwavering love, loyalty, and companionship. They often depend on us for their care and well-being, creating a deep bond of emotional connection. When grieving the loss of a pet, the intensity of emotions can be amplified due to the pure and unconditional love we received from them, as well as the profound sense of responsibility we had towards them.

How has the unconditional love of your pet influenced your life? What did they "teach" you?

Unique Nature of the Relationship:

The relationship with a pet is unique in its simplicity and absence of complexities. Pets often provide a constant source of comfort, joy, and non-judgmental companionship. Unlike human relationships, there is an absence of conflicts, misunderstandings, or complicated dynamics. The loss of a pet can be a profound experience as we mourn the simplicity and pureness of that connection.

Reflect on the profound experience of mourning the pureness and uncomplicated nature of your connection with your beloved pet.

Social Support and Understanding:

Pet grief is often less understood or validated by society compared to human loss. Many may not fully grasp the deep bond between a pet and their owner, leading to feelings of isolation and a lack of empathetic support. However, connecting with pet loss support groups or others who have shared a similar loss can offer much-needed solace and understanding.

Reflect on challenges you have had to to find support. Do you feel others fully understand the bond you had?

<u>Unique Circumstances of the Loss:</u>

The loss of a pet can happen in many ways—through natural causes, accidents, illness, or the difficult decision of euthanasia. These situations often bring emotional challenges, and the decisions made during end-of-life care can lead to feelings of guilt or self-doubt, adding complexity to your grief.

Reflect on any feelings of guilt or self-doubt that may have come up in your unique circumstances.

Silent Grief and Disenfranchised Loss:

Pet grief is often called "silent grief" or "disenfranchised grief" because it isn't always acknowledged or recognized by others. The loss of a pet may not be seen as significant, leaving you without the formal rituals or support systems that typically help in the grieving process. This can make it difficult to express your grief and find validation for your feelings.

Reflect on the impact of this silence. Consider alternate options for comfort and support, such as pet loss communities or personal rituals.

Validate & Acknowledge the Loss

Validating the loss of a pet is a big step in the grieving process, both personally and socially. Pets often occupy a unique and significant place in our lives, offering unconditional love, companionship, and a sense of security like no one else When a pet passes away, the grief experienced can be profound, similar to the loss of a human loved one. However, this grief is sometimes overlooked or minimized by society, which can lead to further emotional pain and isolation for the grieving individual.

Personal Acknowledgment

- Emotional Processing: Personally acknowledging the loss of your pet is essential for healthily processing your grief. Grief that is not fully acknowledged can lead to suppressed emotions, which may manifest later as anxiety, depression, or other mental health issues. By allowing yourself to fully feel and express your emotions, you create space for healing and begin to process the loss in a meaningful way.

- Validation of Your Bond: Your pet was likely a beloved member of your family, and acknowledging their loss validates the bond you shared. This validation is an important part of honouring your pet's memory and recognizing the impact they had on your life. It allows you to cherish the good times and gives you permission to grieve the void left by their absence.

Validate & Acknowledge the Loss

Social Acknowledgment

- Reducing Isolation: Grieving the loss of a pet can sometimes feel isolating, especially if those around you do not recognize the depth of your loss. Social acknowledgment—whether from friends, family, or a wider community—helps to normalize your feelings and reduce this sense of isolation. When others acknowledge your grief, it can be a powerful affirmation that your loss is real and significant, helping you feel supported and understood.

- Preventing Complicated Grief: When the loss of a pet is not socially acknowledged, it can lead to feelings of shame or guilt about your grief. This lack of recognition can contribute to complicated grief, where the grieving process is prolonged and more intense, making it harder to move forward. On the other hand, when others validate your grief, it can ease the burden and facilitate a more natural healing process.

- Promoting Healthy Coping: Social acknowledgment also encourages healthy coping mechanisms. When your grief is validated by others, it becomes easier to express your emotions openly, seek support, and engage in rituals or activities that help you process the loss. This can include talking about your pet, sharing memories, or participating in memorial activities, all of which are important steps in healing.

Validate & Acknowledge the Loss

Potential Impact of Not Recognizing the Loss

- Suppressed Emotions: Failing to acknowledge the loss of a pet, either personally or socially, can lead to suppressed emotions. These unexpressed feelings may eventually surface in other ways, such as chronic stress, anger, or even physical symptoms like headaches or fatigue. Suppressed grief can also interfere with your ability to fully engage in life, leaving you feeling stuck or emotionally numb.

- Complicated Grief and Depression: Without acknowledgment, there is a risk of developing complicated grief, where the sadness and pain of loss become overwhelming and persist for an extended period. This can lead to depression, feelings of worthlessness, or a sense of hopelessness. The inability to move through the stages of grief can also prevent you from finding closure and continuing to live fully.

Validate & Acknowledge the Loss

Potential Impact of Not Recognizing the Loss

- Impact on Future Relationships: Not recognizing the loss of a pet can also affect your ability to form future relationships, whether with new pets or people. Unresolved grief can create barriers to bonding with others, as you may subconsciously avoid forming attachments out of fear of experiencing similar pain again.

Validating the loss of a pet—both personally and socially—is vital for emotional well-being and healing. Acknowledgment allows you to process your grief, honour your pet's memory, and eventually find peace.

"Remember, their spirits continue to live on in our
hearts and the legacy they leave behind."
- Matthew McConaughey

What made your pet unique? Think about specific traits, habits, or quirks that made your pet special. What were the little things they did that always made you smile? How did their personality shine through in everyday moments?

Write a list of your pet's unique characteristics, creating a "personality profile" for your pet, capturing their essence in everyday words.

<u>How did your pet enrich your life?</u>
Think about the ways your pet brought joy, comfort, and companionship into your life. What are some of the most meaningful experiences or milestones you shared together?

Write a letter to your pet, expressing your gratitude for the joy and love they brought into your life. Include specific examples of moments when they made a difference, big or small.

What were your favourite shared activities?

Reflect on the activities you and your pet enjoyed together, whether it was daily walks, playtime, or simply sitting quietly together. How did these moments strengthen your bond?

Create a "memory map" by drawing or listing the places and activities you and your pet enjoyed most. As you work on this, revisit those places in your mind and relive the happiness you felt.

<u>What lessons did your pet teach you?</u>
Pets often teach us valuable lessons about love, patience, living in the moment, non-judgement and forgiveness. What life lessons did your pet impart to you during their time with you?

Write down the lessons you learned from your pet and how they have impacted your life. Consider how you might carry these lessons forward in your daily life as a way to honor their memory and the impact they had in your life.

<u>How do you want to remember your pet?</u>
Reflect on how you wish to keep your pet's memory alive. What aspects of your pet's life and personality do you want to cherish and celebrate?

Create a personal tribute, such as a photo collage, scrapbook, or a dedicated space in your home where you can keep reminders of your pet. Use this space as a focal point for reflection and remembrance. Make a list of the photos or resources you may use to do this. For example, a digital photo frame.

Memory Jar

Create a memory jar where you can write down individual memories of your pet on slips of paper. Whenever you think of a special moment, write it down and add it to the jar. Over time, this jar will become a cherished collection of your most treasured memories, which you can revisit whenever you need comfort.

"The bond between humans and animals is pure and sacred. When we lose a pet, we mourn the loss of a true friend and companion. But in that loss, we can find strength, resilience, and a deeper appreciation for the joy they brought into our lives."

-Betty White

Self-Care in Grief

Create a Space for Emotions
How can you create a space to honour your emotions without judgment or pressure? A space to be kind to yourself and allow all the different emotions that come with grief to exist without trying to push them away or criticize yourself for feeling a certain way.

Try incorporating mindfulness into your grief journey. Practices like meditation, deep breathing exercises, or mindful walks in nature help by promoting emotional regulation, stress reduction, and enhanced self-awareness. What has worked? Or what are you willing to try?

Healthy and Nurturing Activities
What are some healthy and nurturing things you can do for yourself today? This week? What do you need to do to make it happen?

Self-Care in Grief

Prioritizing self-care for your emotional well-being during grief is crucial. It's an ongoing process that evolves as you go through it. Be open to trying new things, be patient with yourself, and remember the activities or practices that have brought you comfort and peace in the past.

How can you prioritize self-care to nurture your emotional well-being? What has brought you comfort and peace at other times in your life?

Self-Care in Grief

Reflect on whether you've been neglecting aspects of your personal care, such as your grooming habits, exercise routines, or general upkeep. Are you still making time for activities that help you feel good about yourself?

Am I noticing changes in my appearance or daily routines?

Self-Care in Grief

Consider if you've experienced any changes in your health, such as frequent fatigue, forgetfulness, or disruptions in sleep and eating patterns. Are there signs that your body might be struggling due to stress or grief?

How is my physical health responding to my grief?

Self-Care in Grief

Pay attention to your emotional state. Are you feeling more moody, irritable, or withdrawn? Reflect on how your mood has been affecting your interactions with others and your overall well-being.

What emotions have I been experiencing more frequently?

Legacy Projects

Legacy projects offer a meaningful and healing way to cope with the loss of a beloved pet. They provide a sense of purpose during the grieving process, allowing you to channel your love and memories into something tangible. By creating a lasting tribute, you celebrate the joy and companionship your pet brought into your life, while also finding solace in the act of remembrance.

These projects not only help you navigate through grief but also keep the memory of your pet alive in a positive and fulfilling way. Losing a pet can feel like losing a family member—they bring so much joy, laughter, and unconditional love into our lives. It's natural to grieve deeply and important to give yourself time to heal.

Legacy Projects

Questions to ask to get you started
- What type of project feels most meaningful to you?
- Are you interested in crafting or DIY projects?
- Do you have anyone who can support you in this project?
- How much time do you want to dedicate to this project?
- How patient are you with long-term projects? Are quick projects more your style?
- What materials or resources do you already have that could be used?
- What is your approximate budget for a memorial project?

Legacy Projects

Storytelling & Writing
Write a heartfelt story or poem about your pet, capturing their unique personality, special moments, and the impact they had on your life.

Memory Book
Create a special memory book or scrapbook dedicated to your pet. Include photographs, stories, and mementos that capture the unique moments and cherished memories you shared together.

Personalized Jewelry & Keepsakes
Jewelry or keepsakes that symbolize your pet's presence and significance - engraved pendants, keychains, or memorial stones with their name or a special message. Wearing or displaying these items can provide a tangible reminder of your pet's love and companionship.

Memorial Garden or Planting
Design and create a memorial garden in honour of your pet. Choose a dedicated area to plant flowers, shrubs, or even a tree. This living tribute can serve as a peaceful sanctuary and a place for reflection.

Legacy Projects

Commemorative Art

Create a piece of art in memory of your pet. A painting, a sculpture, or a digital artwork that reflects their personality and the bond you shared. Displaying this art in your home can provide comfort and serve as a beautiful tribute to your pet's life.

Donation in Their Name

Consider donating to an animal shelter or a pet-related charity in your pet's name. This act of kindness honours your pet's memory and helps other animals in need. You could also sponsor an animal at a local shelter as a living tribute to your beloved companion.

Custom Pet Portrait

Commission a custom portrait of your pet from a local artist or an online service. This portrait can capture the essence of your pet and serve as a lasting keepsake.

After the Loss

The loss of a beloved pet is a deeply emotional experience, and the journey through grief is unique. As time passes, you may begin to think about what comes next. It's important to approach this process with care and consideration, especially when it comes to long-term healing and the idea of welcoming a new pet into your life.

As you heal, it's natural to begin creating new routines and habits that honor your pet's memory while allowing space for new experiences. Here's how to approach it:

Gradually Adjust Daily Habits
Often we have routines that revolve around our pets—whether it's morning walks, feeding times, or play sessions. After a loss, these routines can feel empty and difficult to adjust, even if there are other pets to continue caring for.

Try: Gradually modifying these routines may help to ease the transition.If you used to walk your dog every morning, you might continue the walk but take a different route or invite a friend along. This honours the memory of your pet while allowing you to move forward.

After the Loss

Introduce New Activities.
Exploring new hobbies or activities can help fill the space left by your pet's absence. Whether it's volunteering at an animal shelter, taking up a new exercise routine, pet sitting, dog walking for a friend, or pursuing a creative project, these activities can bring positive energy into your life.

Try: New activities may provide a sense of purpose and joy, helping you to focus on the present and future. They also offer a way to channel the love and care you had for your pet into something new and meaningful.

Balance Remembrance with New Experiences.
While it's important to keep your pet's memory alive, it's also healthy to allow yourself to embrace new experiences and relationships. This doesn't mean forgetting your pet but rather integrating their memory into a broader, ongoing life story.

Try: Balancing remembrance with new experiences ensures that your pet's legacy remains a positive and uplifting part of your life. It allows you to move forward without feeling guilty or like you're leaving your pet behind.

Considering a New Pet

After the death of a pet, you may eventually think about bringing a new animal into your life. It's important to approach this decision with care, ensuring that the time is right for both you and the new pet.

Take Your Time. There is no right time or prescribed waiting period. However, give yourself space to fully grieve and process your previous pet. This will ensure your decision to adopt a new pet is made with a clear and open heart.

Recognize the New Relationship. When you do decide to bring a new pet into your home, take a moment to recognize that this is a new and separate relationship. Your new pet is not a replacement but a new friend who will create their own special place in your heart.

Considering a New Pet

Ensure Readiness. Before adopting a new pet, check in with yourself to make sure you're truly ready. It's about doing what's best for both you and the animal, ensuring a positive experience for everyone involved.

Healing from the loss of a beloved pet takes time, and it's important to move at your own pace. Whether you're honouring your pet's memory, adjusting to new routines, or eventually considering a new pet, these steps are all part of a journey towards healing and growth.

Remember, your pet will always have a special place in your heart, and the love you shared is a lasting legacy that can bring comfort and joy as you move forward in life.

What's Next

Acknowledging these differences between pet grief and people's grief can help individuals navigate their own healing process and seek support tailored to their specific needs. Remember, grieving the loss of a pet is a valid and personal experience, and finding ways to honour the memory of your beloved pet can be an essential part of the healing journey.

Healing

Healing from the loss of a beloved pet takes time and patience. This workbook is intended to be a companion on your journey, offering solace, support, and a safe space to process your emotions. May it provide you with the tools and resources to navigate your grief while honouring the unique bond you shared with your pet.

What's Next

Guidance

Please note that if you find your grief overwhelming or it persists for an extended period, seeking the guidance of a licensed therapist or counsellor is highly recommended. You are not alone, and professionals are available to assist you throughout your healing process.

Regular Check-ins

Take moments to check in with yourself, allowing the ebb and flow of your feelings. Notice the subtle shifts that occur. Keep the conversations alive, both within your heart and with those around you.

Embrace the enduring love and cherished bond you shared with your beloved pet, allowing it to radiate warmth and inspiration throughout your daily life.

Commonly Asked Questions

What can I do if I still feel overwhelming grief months after my pet's passing?

It's important to remember that grief doesn't have a set timeline, and it's okay to still feel deeply sad even months after your pet has passed. If you're finding it difficult to manage these feelings on your own, consider reaching out to a pet loss counsellor, therapist, or confidant who can offer support.

Engaging in regular self-care, participating in memorial activities, and seeking connection with supportive communities can also help ease the ongoing pain.

How do I know if I'm ready for a new pet?

Deciding to bring a new pet into your life is a very personal choice, and it's important to ensure that you've had enough time to grieve your previous pet. Ask yourself if you're looking for a new pet to fill the void left by your loss or if you genuinely feel ready to open your heart to a new companion.

Remember, a new pet is a new chapter, not a replacement. Take your time and make sure you're emotionally prepared to welcome and care for a new pet without feeling guilty or overwhelmed.

Commonly Asked Questions

Is it weird that I am more sad about my dog's death than my dad dying?

No, it's not strange to feel more sad about the loss of a pet than the loss of a family member. Grief is personal, and the intensity of emotions can vary based on the relationships and circumstances involved.

Pets hold a special place in our hearts, providing unconditional love and companionship. Their loss can be deeply felt. Remember that everyone's grief is unique, and there is no right or wrong way to grieve. Allow yourself to process your feelings without judgment and seek support from understanding individuals during this difficult time.

When do I stop feeling sad?

The duration of grief is different for everyone, there is no fixed timeline. Healing takes time, and it's normal to feel sad for a while. Factors such as the bond with your pet and individual coping mechanisms influence the intensity and duration of grief.

It's important to allow yourself to feel and process your emotions without judgment. As you actively engage in the healing process, you may gradually notice the intensity of sadness lessening. However, waves of grief may resurface from time to time.

Seek support, express your feelings, and be patient with yourself. Remember, there is no right or wrong timeline for grief, and it's okay to feel sad.

Additional Options for Support

Seek Support
Reach out to friends, family, or support groups who understand your loss. Consider speaking with a pet loss counsellor if needed.

Professional Support
Some people may seek the assistance of pet loss counsellors or therapists who specialize in grief counselling. Professionals offer guidance and support during the grieving process, helping individuals navigate their emotions and find healthy coping strategies.

Find Supportive Communities
Pet owners often find solace and support in online communities, forums, or social media groups dedicated to pet loss and grief. These platforms provide a space where individuals can share and receive empathy and understanding from others who truly understand.

Confidant with Caregiver Brilliance
A Confidant is a compassionate, personalized support person, offering a space to express emotions, reflect on experiences, and find clarity, helping you work through the complexities of your loss with empathy and understanding.

Keep Reflecting

Thank you for taking the time to care for yourself and explore your emotions.

The following blank pages are here for you to continue your heart journey—take notes as thoughts and feelings arise, and reflect back on this special part of your life.